Survey of Medical School Faculty: Level of Satisfaction with the Medical Library

ISBN 1-57440-172-6

TABLE OF CONTENTS

LIST OF TABLES

THE QUESTIONNAIRE

LIBRARY SATISFACTION

1. **Rate your level of satisfaction with your college's medical library in the following areas:**

    a. **Comfort**

    b. **Hours of access**

    c. **Ability to provide help when needed**

    d. **Skill in developing the information literacy skills of students**

    e. **Quality of the collection of your scholarly pursuits**

    f. **Ease in accessing needed journal articles**

    g. **Interlibrary loan services**

    h. **Expertise of library subject specialists in your field**

    i. **Quality and depth of the information technology available**

LIBRARY SPENDING CHOICES

2. **Imagine yourself running your college library and subject to its budget constraints. Do you think the library should increase spending on:**

    a. **Additional computer workstations and other advanced hardware technologies?**

    b. **Journal subscriptions?**

    c. **Traditional print books?**

    d. **E-books?**

    e. **Librarians?**

    f. **Better facilities?**

RATING SERVICES

3. **Evaluate the following features of your institution's medical library:**

    a. **Range and quality of databases available**

    b. **Range and quality of academic journals available**

    c. **Availability and quality of instruction in library resources**

    d. **Speed and quality of interlibrary loan resources**

e. **Quality of technology instruction available**

f. **Availability and knowledge of library subject specialists in your area**

PARTICIPANTS

Baylor College of Medicine
BCM
BCM/TCH
Brown University
Case Western Cleveland Clinic
Case Western Reserve University
Cincinnati Children's Hospital Medical
    Center/University of Cincinnati
David Geffen School of Medicine at UCLA
Evans
George Washington University
Lake Erie College of Osteopathic Medicine
Medical Univ of SC
Meharry Medical College
Michigan State University
Monash University
Morehouse; LECOM Bradenton
MUSC
Northwestern University
Robert Wood Johnson Univ Hospital
Rush University Medical Center
SUNY Upstate Medical University
TAMHSC
Temple University School of Medicine
Texas A&M College of Medicine
The University of Iowa
Touro University College of Osteopathic
    Medicine-CA
U of MN, Dept. of Psychiatry
U Virginia
UCD
UCLA
UCSF
UMass Medical School
Univ of Illinois College of Med Peoria
University of Arizona
University of Arizona College of Medicine

University of Arizona Health Sciences Center
University of Arizona School of Medicine
University of Auckland
University of CA, Los Angeles
University of Cincinnati
University of Colorado Health Science Center
University of Edinburgh
University of Iowa
University of Iowa Hospitals and Clinics
University of Kentucky Medical College
University of Minnesota Medical School
University of Newcastle
University of Pennsylvania
University of Pittsburgh School of Medicine
University of Texas Health Science Center
University of Texas Houston Medical School
University of Virginia School of Medicine
University of WA, School of Medicine &
    Pharmacology
University of Washington
University of Western Australia
University of Wisconsin-Madison
University Texas Health Science Center San
    Antonio
UNTHSC Fort Worth/TCOM
UNTHSC Texas College of Osteopathic
    Medicine
USC
UT Southwestern Medical Center at Dallas
UTHSCSA
UTMB
UW Madison
UWMF, University of Wisconsin School of
    Medicine and Public Health
Virginia College of Osteopathic Medicine
Westermeyer

CHARACTERISTICS OF THE SAMPLE

Overall sample size was **141**

Country

USA	129
Other	12

Public or Private College Status

Public college	105
Private college	36

Gender

Male	87
Female	54

Tenure Status

Tenured	47
Not tenured but on a tenure track	17
Not tenured and not on a tenure track	77

Number of Years Employed in the Medical Field in a University

Less than 10	33
10-20	53
21-30	30
More than 30	23
Did not answer	2

Age of Participant

30 or under	2
31-39	17
40-49	29
50-59	50
60 or over	43

Annual Income of Participant

Less than $60,000	1
$60,000 to $85,000	17
$85,000 to $125,000	33
$125,000 to $200,000	39
More than $200,000	46
No response	5

Medical Specialty

Neuroscience, Psychiatry, and Psychology	37
Immunology, Biochemistry, Infectious Diseases, and Microbiology	23
Surgery and Anesthesiology	11
Imaging, Pathology, Physiology, and Endocrinology	14
Public Health, Emergency Medicine, Family Practice & Pediatrics	23
Cancer and Oncology	11
Cardiology	10
Urology, Nephrology, OBGYN, and Otolaryngology	11
Other	1

SUMMARY OF MAIN FINDINGS

Library Satisfaction

The overwhelming majority (97.52%) of survey participants are at least "somewhat satisfied" with the comfortability of their college's medical library, with 76.86% of all participants either "satisfied" or "highly satisfied." There is a high level of satisfaction concerning the libraries' hours of access as well, with an identical 97.52% at least "somewhat satisfied." Of the categories polled, the highest level of dissatisfaction was with the quality of the collections of the participants' scholarly pursuits, with 9.24% of all participants either "dissatisfied" or "highly dissatisfied." When broken down by main fields of medicine, "Public Health, Emergency Medicine, and Family Practice & Pediatrics" proved to be the most satisfied in this department, as 36.84% were "highly satisfied," well above the entire sample average of 25.21%. Also registering high marks was "Cancer and Oncology," with 85.72% either "satisfied" or "highly satisfied" with the quality of collections for their scholarly pursuits. These medical fields also reported high levels of satisfaction with the expertise of library subject specialists in their respective fields, with 42.86% of "Cancer and Oncology" being "highly satisfied" (compared to the entire sample mean of 21.74%). On the other end, both "Cardiology" and "Urology, Nephrology, OBGYN, and Otolaryngology" had more than a 10% dissatisfaction fate, the only fields to do so (12.50% for the former, 11.11% for the latter).

Overall, the highest level of satisfaction was with the library's skill in developing the information literacy skills of its students, where 76.52% of participants were either "satisfied" or "highly satisfied" and only 1.74% was "dissatisfied." No one was "highly dissatisfied" in this category.

Library Spending

Most survey participants do not think their libraries should increase spending. The only category for which a majority of the participants would do so was journal subscriptions, as 58.87% of the participants believe their libraries should be spending more in this area. Outside the United States this number is even higher, at 84.62%. As the participant's annual personal income increases, however, the less likely they are to support increased spending on journal subscriptions: all of those making less than $60,000 would increase spending here, as compared to 76.47% of those making $60,000-$85,000, 63.64% of those making $85,000-$125,000, 58.97% of those making $125,000-$200,000, and 47.83% of those making more than $200,000.

In contrast, only 7.8% would increase spending on traditional print books. 13.89% of scholars from private schools would increase spending here, while only 5.71% of public schools would. This percentage increases with participant's age: while no one under the age of 40 would increase spending on traditional print books, 3.45% of those 40-49 would, rising up to 8% for age bracket 50-59, and 13.95% for ages 60 and over. Scholars from both "Immunology, Biochemistry, Infectious Diseases, and Microbiology" and "Imaging, Pathology, Physiology, and Endocrinology" also were more likely than others to support higher print book spending, at 21.74% and 21.43%, respectively, by far the highest percentages of support for all the medical fields.

When asked about e-book spending, however, 35.46% of all participants would like to see the library spending more. This figure is even higher outside the United States, at 46.15%. 46.81% of tenured participants would increase spending on e-books, as compared to 35.06% of those not tenured and not on a tenured track. Only 5.88% of those who are not tenured but are on a tenured track would increase library spending here. Of the medical fields, scholars in "Cardiology" recorded the highest response at 60%.

Only 25.53% of survey participants think their libraries should be spending more on additional computer workstations. However, this figure increases with the age of participant. So while no one under the age of 30 would increase spending in this department, 5.88% of participants ages 31-39 would, rising up to 17.24% for ages 40-49, 28% for ages 50-59, and finally 37.21% for those over the age of 60. "Neuroscience, Psychiatry, and Psychology" was the medical field with the highest approval rate at 37.84%, while only 10% of scholars in "Cardiology" would increase spending on computer workstations.

Only 14.18% would look to increase spending on more librarians, although this number is higher for countries outside the United States, at 23.08%. The split between public and private schools is 12.38% for public and 19.44% for private, and while only 10.34% of men would increase spending on librarians, 20.37% of women would do so. "Imaging, Pathology, Physiology, and Endocrinology" was the medical field with the highest percentage of participants who would increase spending on librarians at 28.57%.

Databases

We asked the survey participants to evaluate the following features of their institution's medical library: a) range and quality of databases available; b) range and quality of academic journals available; c) availability and quality of instruction in library resources; d) speed and quality of interlibrary loan resources; e) quality of technology instruction; and f) availability and knowledge of quality of library subject specialists in the library's area. Their choices were: 1) excellent; 2) good; 3) acceptable; and 4) poor.

Both the range and quality of databases available and the range and quality of academic journals available scored high marks, with 46.83% of participants rating the former category "excellent" and 50% rating the latter the same way. No other category rated higher than 32% with "excellent" responses. Participants outside the United States rated their institutions' range of quality of databases higher (58.33% "excellent") than those participants within the United States (45.61% "excellent"). This split is even at 50-50 for the range and quality of academic journals available, although public and private schools differ here: 52.63% of public schools responded "excellent," as compared to 41.94% of private schools. Furthermore, 9.68% of private schools responded "poor" for this category.

When asked to evaluate the availability and quality of instruction in library resources, private schools tended to be the most polarizing. So while 70.78% of public schools rated their libraries' performances in this area as either "good" or "acceptable," 46.67% of private schools responded "excellent" (26.97% for public) and 10.00% responded "poor" (2.25% for public), leaving just 43.33% for the two middle answers. These were also well above the entire sample averages of 31.93% for "excellent" and 4.20% for "poor." Participants from countries outside the U.S. rated these library functions as either "good" or "excellent" 90.91% of the time, as compared to 72.22% of U.S. participants.

In regards to the speed and quality of interlibrary loan resources, the responses from private schools were again polarizing, as 40.00% rated these services as "excellent" while 13.33% rated them "poor." By comparison, 66.30% of public schools responded in the middle of the pack with either "good" or "acceptable" (46.67% for private). Again, the numbers for private schools were above the entire sample averages of 31.97% for "excellent" and 6.56% for "poor" and these participants responded in a similar fashion to questions concerning the quality of technology instruction and the availability/knowledge/quality of library subject specialists.

Chapter One: Library Satisfaction

Question One: Rate your level of satisfaction concerning the comfort of your college's medical library.

Table 1.1: Rate your level of satisfaction concerning the comfort of your college's medical library.

	Highly Satisfied	Satisfied	Somewhat Satisfied	Dissatisfied	Highly Dissatisfied
Entire Sample	25.62%	51.24%	20.66%	2.48%	0.00%

Table 1.2: Rate your level of satisfaction concerning the comfort of your college's medical library. Broken out by country.

Country	Highly Satisfied	Satisfied	Somewhat Satisfied	Dissatisfied	Highly Dissatisfied
USA	25.00%	51.85%	20.37%	2.78%	0.00%
Other	30.77%	46.15%	23.08%	0.00%	0.00%

Table 1.3: Rate your level of satisfaction concerning the comfort of your college's medical library. Broken out by public or private college status.

Type of College	Highly Satisfied	Satisfied	Somewhat Satisfied	Dissatisfied	Highly Dissatisfied
Public	25.84%	50.56%	20.22%	3.37%	0.00%
Private	25.00%	53.13%	21.88%	0.00%	0.00%

Table 1.4: Rate your level of satisfaction concerning the comfort of your college's medical library. Broken out by age of participant.

Age	Highly Satisfied	Satisfied	Somewhat Satisfied	Dissatisfied	Highly Dissatisfied
30 or under	50.00%	0.00%	0.00%	50.00%	0.00%
31-39	14.29%	71.43%	14.29%	0.00%	0.00%
40-49	28.00%	36.00%	32.00%	4.00%	0.00%
50-59	28.57%	52.38%	16.67%	2.38%	0.00%
60 or over	23.68%	55.26%	21.05%	0.00%	0.00%

Table 1.5: Rate your level of satisfaction concerning the comfort of your college's medical library. Broken out by gender.

Gender	Highly Satisfied	Satisfied	Somewhat Satisfied	Dissatisfied	Highly Dissatisfied
Male	28.00%	46.67%	24.00%	1.33%	0.00%
Female	21.74%	58.70%	15.22%	4.35%	0.00%

Table 1.6: Rate your level of satisfaction concerning the comfort of your college's medical library. Broken out by annual personal income.

Annual Personal Income	Highly Satisfied	Satisfied	Somewhat Satisfied	Dissatisfied	Highly Dissatisfied
Less than $60,000	0.00%	0.00%	100.00%	0.00%	0.00%
$60,000 to $85,000	0.00%	71.43%	28.57%	0.00%	0.00%
$85,000 to $125,000	48.28%	34.48%	13.79%	3.45%	0.00%
$125,000 to 200,000	25.00%	56.25%	15.63%	3.13%	0.00%
More than $200,000	20.00%	57.50%	22.50%	0.00%	0.00%

Table 1.7: Rate your level of satisfaction concerning the comfort of your college's medical library. Broken out by tenure status.

Tenure Status	Highly Satisfied	Satisfied	Somewhat Satisfied	Dissatisfied	Highly Dissatisfied
Tenured	12.82%	58.97%	28.21%	0.00%	0.00%
Not tenured but on a tenure track	15.38%	61.54%	7.69%	15.38%	0.00%
Not tenured and not on a tenure track	34.78%	44.93%	18.84%	1.45%	0.00%

Table 1.8: Rate your level of satisfaction concerning the comfort of your college's medical library. Broken out by main field of medical research.

Main Field of Medical Research	Highly Satisfied	Satisfied	Somewhat Satisfied	Dissatisfied	Highly Dissatisfied
Neuroscience, Psychiatry, and Psychology	20.59%	52.94%	26.47%	0.00%	0.00%
Immunology, Biochemistry, Infectious Diseases, and Microbiology	23.81%	57.14%	14.29%	4.76%	0.00%
Surgery and Anesthesiology	11.11%	55.56%	22.22%	11.11%	0.00%
Imaging, Pathology, Physiology, and Endocrinology	41.67%	16.67%	41.67%	0.00%	0.00%
Public Health, Emergency Medicine, and Family Practice & Pediatrics	52.63%	42.11%	5.26%	0.00%	0.00%
Cancer and Oncology	12.50%	75.00%	12.50%	0.00%	0.00%
Cardiology	25.00%	37.50%	25.00%	12.50%	0.00%
Urology, Nephrology, OBGYN, and Otolaryngology	0.00%	80.00%	20.00%	0.00%	0.00%

Question Two: Rate your level of satisfaction concerning your college's medical library's hours of access.

Table 1.9: Rate your level of satisfaction concerning your college's medical library's hours of access.

	Highly Satisfied	Satisfied	Somewhat Satisfied	Dissatisfied	Highly Dissatisfied
Entire Sample	24.79%	55.37%	17.36%	2.48%	0.00%

Table 1.10: Rate your level of satisfaction concerning your college's medical library's hours of access. Broken out by country.

Country	Highly Satisfied	Satisfied	Somewhat Satisfied	Dissatisfied	Highly Dissatisfied
USA	25.00%	53.70%	18.52%	2.78%	0.00%
Other	23.08%	69.23%	7.69%	0.00%	0.00%

Table 1.11: Rate your level of satisfaction concerning your college's medical library's hours of access. Broken out by public or private college status.

Type of College	Highly Satisfied	Satisfied	Somewhat Satisfied	Dissatisfied	Highly Dissatisfied
Public	24.72%	55.06%	16.85%	3.37%	0.00%
Private	25.00%	56.25%	18.75%	0.00%	0.00%

Table 1.12: Rate your level of satisfaction concerning your college's medical library's hours of access. Broken out by age of participant.

Age	Highly Satisfied	Satisfied	Somewhat Satisfied	Dissatisfied	Highly Dissatisfied
30 or under	50.00%	0.00%	50.00%	0.00%	0.00%
31-39	0.00%	85.71%	14.29%	0.00%	0.00%
40-49	28.00%	44.00%	24.00%	4.00%	0.00%
50-59	28.57%	52.38%	14.29%	4.76%	0.00%
60 or over	26.32%	57.89%	15.79%	0.00%	0.00%

Survey of Medical School Faculty: Level of Satisfaction with the Medical Library

Table 1.13: Rate your level of satisfaction concerning your college's medical library's hours of access. Broken out by gender.

Gender	Highly Satisfied	Satisfied	Somewhat Satisfied	Dissatisfied	Highly Dissatisfied
Male	26.67%	52.00%	18.67%	2.67%	0.00%
Female	21.74%	60.87%	15.22%	2.17%	0.00%

Table 1.14: Rate your level of satisfaction concerning your college's medical library's hours of access. Broken out by annual personal income.

Annual Personal Income	Highly Satisfied	Satisfied	Somewhat Satisfied	Dissatisfied	Highly Dissatisfied
Less than $60,000	0.00%	0.00%	100.00%	0.00%	0.00%
$60,000 to $85,000	7.14%	71.43%	21.43%	0.00%	0.00%
$85,000 to $125,000	41.38%	44.83%	13.79%	0.00%	0.00%
$125,000 to 200,000	21.88%	59.38%	12.50%	6.25%	0.00%
More than $200,000	22.50%	60.00%	17.50%	0.00%	0.00%

Table 1.15: Rate your level of satisfaction concerning your college's medical library's hours of access. Broken out by tenure status.

Tenure Status	Highly Satisfied	Satisfied	Somewhat Satisfied	Dissatisfied	Highly Dissatisfied
Tenured	17.95%	64.10%	17.95%	0.00%	0.00%
Not tenured but on a tenure track	7.69%	61.54%	23.08%	7.69%	0.00%
Not tenured and not on a tenure track	31.88%	49.28%	15.94%	2.90%	0.00%

23

Table 1.16: Rate your level of satisfaction concerning your college's medical library's hours of access. Broken out by main field of medical research.

Main Field of Medical Research	Highly Satisfied	Satisfied	Somewhat Satisfied	Dissatisfied	Highly Dissatisfied
Neuroscience, Psychiatry, and Psychology	29.41%	50.00%	20.59%	0.00%	0.00%
Immunology, Biochemistry, Infectious Diseases, and Microbiology	23.81%	57.14%	14.29%	4.76%	0.00%
Surgery and Anesthesiology	11.11%	55.56%	33.33%	0.00%	0.00%
Imaging, Pathology, Physiology, and Endocrinology	25.00%	41.67%	25.00%	8.33%	0.00%
Public Health, Emergency Medicine, and Family Practice & Pediatrics	42.11%	52.63%	5.26%	0.00%	0.00%
Cancer and Oncology	12.50%	75.00%	12.50%	0.00%	0.00%
Cardiology	25.00%	37.50%	25.00%	12.50%	0.00%
Urology, Nephrology, OBGYN, and Otolaryngology	0.00%	90.00%	10.00%	0.00%	0.00%

Question Three: Rate your level of satisfaction concerning your college's medical library's ability to provide help when needed.

Table 1.17: Rate your level of satisfaction concerning your college's medical library's ability to provide help when needed.

	Highly Satisfied	Satisfied	Somewhat Satisfied	Dissatisfied	Highly Dissatisfied
Entire Sample	26.89%	48.74%	20.17%	3.36%	0.84%

Table 1.18: Rate your level of satisfaction concerning your college's medical library's ability to provide help when needed. Broken out by country.

Country	Highly Satisfied	Satisfied	Somewhat Satisfied	Dissatisfied	Highly Dissatisfied
USA	27.36%	48.11%	19.81%	3.77%	0.94%
Other	23.08%	53.85%	23.08%	0.00%	0.00%

Table 1.19: Rate your level of satisfaction concerning your college's medical library's ability to provide help when needed. Broken out by public or private college status.

Type of College	Highly Satisfied	Satisfied	Somewhat Satisfied	Dissatisfied	Highly Dissatisfied
Public	28.74%	49.43%	17.24%	4.60%	0.00%
Private	21.88%	46.88%	28.13%	0.00%	3.13%

Table 1.20: Rate your level of satisfaction concerning your college's medical library's ability to provide help when needed. Broken out by age of participant.

Age	Highly Satisfied	Satisfied	Somewhat Satisfied	Dissatisfied	Highly Dissatisfied
30 or under	50.00%	0.00%	50.00%	0.00%	0.00%
31-39	21.43%	50.00%	28.57%	0.00%	0.00%
40-49	28.00%	48.00%	12.00%	8.00%	4.00%
50-59	25.00%	47.50%	22.50%	5.00%	0.00%
60 or over	28.95%	52.63%	18.42%	0.00%	0.00%

Table 1.21: Rate your level of satisfaction concerning your college's medical library's ability to provide help when needed. Broken out by gender.

Gender	Highly Satisfied	Satisfied	Somewhat Satisfied	Dissatisfied	Highly Dissatisfied
Male	24.32%	54.05%	18.92%	2.70%	0.00%
Female	31.11%	40.00%	22.22%	4.44%	2.22%

Table 1.22: Rate your level of satisfaction concerning your college's medical library's ability to provide help when needed. Broken out by annual personal income.

Annual Personal Income	Highly Satisfied	Satisfied	Somewhat Satisfied	Dissatisfied	Highly Dissatisfied
Less than $60,000	0.00%	0.00%	100.00%	0.00%	0.00%
$60,000 to $85,000	21.43%	42.86%	35.71%	0.00%	0.00%
$85,000 to $125,000	41.38%	41.38%	13.79%	3.45%	0.00%
$125,000 to 200,000	30.00%	53.33%	13.33%	3.33%	0.00%
More than $200,000	17.50%	57.50%	20.00%	2.50%	2.50%

Table 1.23: Rate your level of satisfaction concerning your college's medical library's ability to provide help when needed. Broken out by tenure status.

Tenure Status	Highly Satisfied	Satisfied	Somewhat Satisfied	Dissatisfied	Highly Dissatisfied
Tenured	15.38%	66.67%	17.95%	0.00%	0.00%
Not tenured but on a tenure track	15.38%	46.15%	30.77%	7.69%	0.00%
Not tenured and not on a tenure track	35.82%	38.81%	19.40%	4.48%	1.49%

Table 1.24: Rate your level of satisfaction concerning your college's medical library's ability to provide help when needed. Broken out by main field of medical research.

Main Field of Medical Research	Highly Satisfied	Satisfied	Somewhat Satisfied	Dissatisfied	Highly Dissatisfied
Neuroscience, Psychiatry, and Psychology	26.47%	50.00%	20.59%	2.94%	0.00%
Immunology, Biochemistry, Infectious Diseases, and Microbiology	20.00%	70.00%	5.00%	5.00%	0.00%
Surgery and Anesthesiology	11.11%	44.44%	44.44%	0.00%	0.00%
Imaging, Pathology, Physiology, and Endocrinology	25.00%	16.67%	50.00%	8.33%	0.00%
Public Health, Emergency Medicine, and Family Practice & Pediatrics	50.00%	50.00%	0.00%	0.00%	0.00%
Cancer and Oncology	37.50%	37.50%	25.00%	0.00%	0.00%
Cardiology	25.00%	25.00%	37.50%	12.50%	0.00%
Urology, Nephrology, OBGYN, and Otolaryngology	10.00%	70.00%	10.00%	0.00%	10.00%

Question Four: Rate your level of satisfaction concerning your college's medical library's skill in developing the information literacy skills of students.

Table 1.25: Rate your level of satisfaction concerning your college's medical library's skill in developing the information literacy skills of students.

	Highly Satisfied	Satisfied	Somewhat Satisfied	Dissatisfied	Highly Dissatisfied
Entire Sample	22.61%	53.91%	21.74%	1.74%	0.00%

Table 1.26: Rate your level of satisfaction concerning your college's medical library's skill in developing the information literacy skills of students. Broken out by country.

Country	Highly Satisfied	Satisfied	Somewhat Satisfied	Dissatisfied	Highly Dissatisfied
USA	22.33%	53.40%	22.33%	1.94%	0.00%
Other	25.00%	58.33%	16.67%	0.00%	0.00%

Table 1.27: Rate your level of satisfaction concerning your college's medical library's skill in developing the information literacy skills of students. Broken out by public or private college status.

Type of College	Highly Satisfied	Satisfied	Somewhat Satisfied	Dissatisfied	Highly Dissatisfied
Public	21.43%	53.57%	22.62%	2.38%	0.00%
Private	25.81%	54.84%	19.35%	0.00%	0.00%

Table 1.28: Rate your level of satisfaction concerning your college's medical library's skill in developing the information literacy skills of students. Broken out by age of participant.

Age	Highly Satisfied	Satisfied	Somewhat Satisfied	Dissatisfied	Highly Dissatisfied
30 or under	50.00%	0.00%	50.00%	0.00%	0.00%
31-39	18.18%	54.55%	27.27%	0.00%	0.00%
40-49	20.83%	54.17%	25.00%	0.00%	0.00%
50-59	14.63%	58.54%	21.95%	4.88%	0.00%
60 or over	32.43%	51.35%	16.22%	0.00%	0.00%

Survey of Medical School Faculty: Level of Satisfaction with the Medical Library

Table 1.29:   Rate your level of satisfaction concerning your college's medical library's skill in developing the information literacy skills of students. Broken out by gender.

Gender	Highly Satisfied	Satisfied	Somewhat Satisfied	Dissatisfied	Highly Dissatisfied
Male	26.03%	53.42%	17.81%	2.74%	0.00%
Female	16.67%	54.76%	28.57%	0.00%	0.00%

Table 1.30:   Rate your level of satisfaction concerning your college's medical library's skill in developing the information literacy skills of students. Broken out by annual personal income.

Annual Personal Income	Highly Satisfied	Satisfied	Somewhat Satisfied	Dissatisfied	Highly Dissatisfied
Less than $60,000	0.00%	100.00%	0.00%	0.00%	0.00%
$60,000 to $85,000	15.38%	46.15%	38.46%	0.00%	0.00%
$85,000 to $125,000	44.44%	37.04%	18.52%	0.00%	0.00%
$125,000 to 200,000	20.69%	65.52%	13.79%	0.00%	0.00%
More than $200,000	12.50%	62.50%	22.50%	2.50%	0.00%

Table 1.31:   Rate your level of satisfaction concerning your college's medical library's skill in developing the information literacy skills of students. Broken out by tenure status.

Tenure Status	Highly Satisfied	Satisfied	Somewhat Satisfied	Dissatisfied	Highly Dissatisfied
Tenured	10.53%	57.89%	31.58%	0.00%	0.00%
Not tenured but on a tenure track	25.00%	50.00%	25.00%	0.00%	0.00%
Not tenured and not on a tenure track	29.23%	52.31%	15.38%	3.08%	0.00%

Table 1.32: Rate your level of satisfaction concerning your college's medical library's skill in developing the information literacy skills of students. Broken out by main field of medical research.

Main Field of Medical Research	Highly Satisfied	Satisfied	Somewhat Satisfied	Dissatisfied	Highly Dissatisfied
Neuroscience, Psychiatry, and Psychology	18.75%	56.25%	`21.87%	3.12%	0.00%
Immunology, Biochemistry, Infectious Diseases, and Microbiology	21.05%	57.89%	15.79%	5.26%	0.00%
Surgery and Anesthesiology	11.11%	44.44%	44.44%	0.00%	0.00%
Imaging, Pathology, Physiology, and Endocrinology	18.18%	36.36%	45.45%	0.00%	0.00%
Public Health, Emergency Medicine, and Family Practice & Pediatrics	50.00%	50.00%	0.00%	0.00%	0.00%
Cancer and Oncology	25.00%	50.00%	25.00%	0.00%	0.00%
Cardiology	12.50%	50.00%	37.50%	0.00%	0.00%
Urology, Nephrology, OBGYN, and Otolaryngology	10.00%	80.00%	10.00%	0.00%	0.00%

Question Five: Rate your level of satisfaction concerning the quality of the collection for your scholarly pursuits at your college's medical library.

Table 1.33: Rate your level of satisfaction concerning the quality of the collection for your scholarly pursuits at your college's medical library.

	Highly Satisfied	Satisfied	Somewhat Satisfied	Dissatisfied	Highly Dissatisfied
Entire Sample	25.21%	42.86%	22.69%	7.56%	1.68%

Table 1.34: Rate your level of satisfaction concerning the quality of the collection for your scholarly pursuits at your college's medical library. Broken out by country.

Country	Highly Satisfied	Satisfied	Somewhat Satisfied	Dissatisfied	Highly Dissatisfied
USA	24.53%	43.40%	22.64%	7.55%	1.89%
Other	30.77%	38.46%	23.08%	7.69%	0.00%

Table 1.35: Rate your level of satisfaction concerning the quality of the collection for your scholarly pursuits at your college's medical library. Broken out by public or private college status.

Type of College	Highly Satisfied	Satisfied	Somewhat Satisfied	Dissatisfied	Highly Dissatisfied
Public	25.84%	43.82%	25.84%	4.49%	0.00%
Private	23.33%	40.00%	13.33%	16.67%	6.67%

Table 1.36: Rate your level of satisfaction concerning the quality of the collection for your scholarly pursuits at your college's medical library. Broken out by age of participant.

Age	Highly Satisfied	Satisfied	Somewhat Satisfied	Dissatisfied	Highly Dissatisfied
30 or under	50.00%	0.00%	50.00%	0.00%	0.00%
31-39	0.00%	92.86%	7.14%	0.00%	0.00%
40-49	29.17%	29.17%	33.33%	8.33%	0.00%
50-59	28.57%	40.48%	19.05%	9.52%	2.38%
60 or over	27.03%	37.84%	24.32%	8.11%	2.70%

Table 1.37: Rate your level of satisfaction concerning the quality of the collection for your scholarly pursuits at your college's medical library. Broken out by gender.

Gender	Highly Satisfied	Satisfied	Somewhat Satisfied	Dissatisfied	Highly Dissatisfied
Male	25.33%	45.33%	18.67%	9.33%	1.33%
Female	25.00%	38.64%	29.55%	4.55%	2.27%

Table 1.38: Rate your level of satisfaction concerning the quality of the collection for your scholarly pursuits at your college's medical library. Broken out by annual personal income.

Annual Personal Income	Highly Satisfied	Satisfied	Somewhat Satisfied	Dissatisfied	Highly Dissatisfied
Less than $60,000	0.00%	100.00%	0.00%	0.00%	0.00%
$60,000 to $85,000	7.14%	57.14%	35.71%	0.00%	0.00%
$85,000 to $125,000	32.14%	28.57%	25.00%	14.29%	0.00%
$125,000 to 200,000	28.13%	46.88%	12.50%	6.25%	6.25%
More than $200,000	25.64%	46.15%	23.08%	5.13%	0.00%

Table 1.39: Rate your level of satisfaction concerning the quality of the collection for your scholarly pursuits at your college's medical library. Broken out by tenure status.

Tenure Status	Highly Satisfied	Satisfied	Somewhat Satisfied	Dissatisfied	Highly Dissatisfied
Tenured	16.22%	48.65%	32.43%	2.70%	0.00%
Not tenured but on a tenure track	0.00%	69.23%	30.77%	0.00%	0.00%
Not tenured and not on a tenure track	34.78%	34.78%	15.94%	11.59%	2.90%

Table 1.40: Rate your level of satisfaction concerning the quality of the collection for your scholarly pursuits at your college's medical library. Broken out by main field of medical research.

Main Field of Medical Research	Highly Satisfied	Satisfied	Somewhat Satisfied	Dissatisfied	Highly Dissatisfied
Neuroscience, Psychiatry, and Psychology	29.41%	32.35%	29.41%	5.88%	2.94%
Immunology, Biochemistry, Infectious Diseases, and Microbiology	20.00%	55.00%	15.00%	5.00%	5.00%
Surgery and Anesthesiology	22.22%	33.33%	44.44%	0.00%	0.00%
Imaging, Pathology, Physiology, and Endocrinology	25.00%	33.33%	16.67%	25.00%	0.00%
Public Health, Emergency Medicine, and Family Practice & Pediatrics	36.84%	47.37%	15.79%	0.00%	0.00%
Cancer and Oncology	14.29%	71.43%	14.29%	0.00%	0.00%
Cardiology	25.00%	37.50%	25.00%	12.50%	0.00%
Urology, Nephrology, OBGYN, and Otolaryngology	10.00%	50.00%	20.00%	20.00%	0.00%

Question Six: Rate your level of satisfaction concerning the ease in asccessing needed journal articles at your college's medical library.

Table 1.41: Rate your level of satisfaction concerning the ease in accessing needed journal articles at your college's medical library.

	Highly Satisfied	Satisfied	Somewhat Satisfied	Dissatisfied	Highly Dissatisfied
Entire Sample	34.17%	41.67%	19.17%	4.17%	0.83%

Table 1.42: Rate your level of satisfaction concerning the ease in accessing needed journal articles at your college's medical library. Broken out by country.

Country	Highly Satisfied	Satisfied	Somewhat Satisfied	Dissatisfied	Highly Dissatisfied
USA	34.58%	41.12%	19.63%	3.74%	0.93%
Other	30.77%	46.15%	15.38%	7.69%	0.00%

Table 1.43: Rate your level of satisfaction concerning the ease in accessing needed journal articles at your college's medical library. Broken out by public or private college status.

Type of College	Highly Satisfied	Satisfied	Somewhat Satisfied	Dissatisfied	Highly Dissatisfied
Public	37.08%	40.45%	16.85%	5.62%	0.00%
Private	25.81%	45.16%	25.81%	0.00%	3.23%

Table 1.44: Rate your level of satisfaction concerning the ease in accessing needed journal articles at your college's medical library. Broken out by age of participant.

Age	Highly Satisfied	Satisfied	Somewhat Satisfied	Dissatisfied	Highly Dissatisfied
30 or under	50.00%	0.00%	50.00%	0.00%	0.00%
31-39	14.29%	78.57%	7.14%	0.00%	0.00%
40-49	48.00%	32.00%	20.00%	0.00%	0.00%
50-59	28.57%	35.71%	26.19%	7.14%	2.38%
60 or over	37.84%	43.24%	13.51%	5.41%	0.00%

Table 1.45: Rate your level of satisfaction concerning the ease in accessing needed journal articles at your college's medical library. Broken out by gender.

Gender	Highly Satisfied	Satisfied	Somewhat Satisfied	Dissatisfied	Highly Dissatisfied
Male	34.67%	44.00%	14.67%	6.67%	0.00%
Female	33.33%	37.78%	26.67%	0.00%	2.22%

Table 1.46: Rate your level of satisfaction concerning the ease in accessing needed journal articles at your college's medical library. Broken out by annual personal income.

Annual Personal Income	Highly Satisfied	Satisfied	Somewhat Satisfied	Dissatisfied	Highly Dissatisfied
Less than $60,000	100.00%	0.00%	0.00%	0.00%	0.00%
$60,000 to $85,000	14.29%	57.14%	28.57%	0.00%	0.00%
$85,000 to $125,000	41.38%	31.03%	24.14%	3.45%	0.00%
$125,000 to 200,000	34.38%	46.88%	15.63%	0.00%	3.13%
More than $200,000	35.90%	43.59%	12.82%	7.69%	0.00%

Table 1.47: Rate your level of satisfaction concerning the ease in accessing needed journal articles at your college's medical library. Broken out by tenure status.

Tenure Status	Highly Satisfied	Satisfied	Somewhat Satisfied	Dissatisfied	Highly Dissatisfied
Tenured	28.95%	47.37%	21.05%	2.63%	0.00%
Not tenured but on a tenure track	30.77%	53.85%	15.38%	0.00%	0.00%
Not tenured and not on a tenure track	37.68%	36.23%	18.84%	5.80%	1.45%

Table 1.48:   Rate your level of satisfaction concerning the ease in accessing needed journal articles at your college's medical library. Broken out by main field of medical research.

Main Field of Medical Research	Highly Satisfied	Satisfied	Somewhat Satisfied	Dissatisfied	Highly Dissatisfied
Neuroscience, Psychiatry, and Psychology	35.29%	44.12%	11.76%	5.88%	2.94%
Immunology, Biochemistry, Infectious Diseases, and Microbiology	38.10%	47.62%	9.52%	4.76%	0.00%
Surgery and Anesthesiology	22.22%	22.22%	44.44%	11.11%	0.00%
Imaging, Pathology, Physiology, and Endocrinology	16.67%	41.67%	33.33%	8.33%	0.00%
Public Health, Emergency Medicine, and Family Practice & Pediatrics	42.11%	36.84%	21.05%	0.00%	0.00%
Cancer and Oncology	42.86%	57.14%	0.00%	0.00%	0.00%
Cardiology	50.00%	25.00%	25.00%	0.00%	0.00%
Urology, Nephrology, OBGYN, and Otolaryngology	20.00%	50.00%	30.00%	0.00%	0.00%

Question Seven: Rate your level of satisfaction concerning your college medical library's interlibrary loan resources.

Table 1.49: Rate your level of satisfaction concerning your college medical library's interlibrary loan resources.

	Highly Satisfied	Satisfied	Somewhat Satisfied	Dissatisfied	Highly Dissatisfied
Entire Sample	36.44%	38.14%	20.34%	4.24%	0.85%

Table 1.50: Rate your level of satisfaction concerning your college medical library's interlibrary loan resources. Broken out by country.

Country	Highly Satisfied	Satisfied	Somewhat Satisfied	Dissatisfied	Highly Dissatisfied
USA	37.14%	36.19%	20.95%	4.76%	0.95%
Other	30.77%	53.85%	15.38%	0.00%	0.00%

Table 1.51: Rate your level of satisfaction concerning your college medical library's interlibrary loan resources. Broken out by public or private college status.

Type of College	Highly Satisfied	Satisfied	Somewhat Satisfied	Dissatisfied	Highly Dissatisfied
Public	37.08%	39.33%	20.22%	3.37%	0.00%
Private	34.48%	34.48%	20.69%	6.90%	3.45%

Table 1.52: Rate your level of satisfaction concerning your college medical library's interlibrary loan resources. Broken out by age of participant.

Age	Highly Satisfied	Satisfied	Somewhat Satisfied	Dissatisfied	Highly Dissatisfied
30 or under	50.00%	0.00%	50.00%	0.00%	0.00%
31-39	23.08%	61.54%	15.38%	0.00%	0.00%
40-49	33.33%	37.50%	20.83%	4.17%	4.17%
50-59	40.48%	30.95%	21.43%	7.14%	0.00%
60 or over	37.84%	40.54%	18.92%	2.70%	0.00%

Table 1.53: Rate your level of satisfaction concerning your college medical library's interlibrary loan resources. Broken out by gender.

Gender	Highly Satisfied	Satisfied	Somewhat Satisfied	Dissatisfied	Highly Dissatisfied
Male	33.78%	44.59%	16.22%	5.41%	0.00%
Female	40.91%	27.27%	27.27%	2.27%	2.27%

Table 1.54: Rate your level of satisfaction concerning your college medical library's interlibrary loan resources. Broken out by annual personal income.

Annual Personal Income	Highly Satisfied	Satisfied	Somewhat Satisfied	Dissatisfied	Highly Dissatisfied
Less than $60,000	0.00%	100.00%	0.00%	0.00%	0.00%
$60,000 to $85,000	21.43%	50.00%	28.57%	0.00%	0.00%
$85,000 to $125,000	39.29%	35.71%	25.00%	0.00%	0.00%
$125,000 to 200,000	46.88%	34.38%	12.50%	6.25%	0.00%
More than $200,000	34.21%	39.47%	18.42%	5.26%	2.63%

Table 1.55: Rate your level of satisfaction concerning your college medical library's interlibrary loan resources. Broken out by tenure status.

Tenure Status	Highly Satisfied	Satisfied	Somewhat Satisfied	Dissatisfied	Highly Dissatisfied
Tenured	29.73%	43.24%	24.32%	2.70%	0.00%
Not tenured but on a tenure track	25.00%	50.00%	16.67%	8.33%	0.00%
Not tenured and not on a tenure track	42.03%	33.33%	18.84%	4.35%	1.45%

Table 1.56:   Rate your level of satisfaction concerning your college medical library's interlibrary loan resources. Broken out by main field of medical research.

Main Field of Medical Research	Highly Satisfied	Satisfied	Somewhat Satisfied	Dissatisfied	Highly Dissatisfied
Neuroscience, Psychiatry, and Psychology	41.18%	35.29%	17.65%	5.88%	0.00%
Immunology, Biochemistry, Infectious Diseases, and Microbiology	25.00%	55.00%	15.00%	5.00%	0.00%
Surgery and Anesthesiology	22.22%	33.33%	44.44%	0.00%	0.00%
Imaging, Pathology, Physiology, and Endocrinology	33.33%	33.33%	33.33%	0.00%	0.00%
Public Health, Emergency Medicine, and Family Practice & Pediatrics	47.37%	36.84%	15.79%	0.00%	0.00%
Cancer and Oncology	42.86%	42.86%	14.29%	0.00%	0.00%
Cardiology	50.00%	12.50%	12.50%	25.00%	0.00%
Urology, Nephrology, OBGYN, and Otolaryngology	22.22%	44.44%	22.22%	0.00%	11.11%

Question Eight: Rate your level of satisfaction concerning the expertise of library subject specialists in your field at your college's medical library.

Table 1.57:   Rate your level of satisfaction concerning the expertise of library subject specialists in your field at your college's medical library.

	Highly Satisfied	Satisfied	Somewhat Satisfied	Dissatisfied	Highly Dissatisfied
Entire Sample	21.74%	41.74%	29.57%	5.22%	1.74%

Table 1.58:   Rate your level of satisfaction concerning the expertise of library subject specialists in your field at your college's medical library. Broken out by country.

Country	Highly Satisfied	Satisfied	Somewhat Satisfied	Dissatisfied	Highly Dissatisfied
USA	21.57%	42.16%	29.41%	5.88%	0.98%
Other	23.08%	38.46%	30.77%	0.00%	7.69%

Table 1.59:   Rate your level of satisfaction concerning the expertise of library subject specialists in your field at your college's medical library. Broken out by public or private college status.

Type of College	Highly Satisfied	Satisfied	Somewhat Satisfied	Dissatisfied	Highly Dissatisfied
Public	22.09%	46.51%	26.74%	3.49%	1.16%
Private	20.69%	27.59%	37.93%	10.34%	3.45%

Table 1.60:   Rate your level of satisfaction concerning the expertise of library subject specialists in your field at your college's medical library. Broken out by age of participant.

Age	Highly Satisfied	Satisfied	Somewhat Satisfied	Dissatisfied	Highly Dissatisfied
30 or under	0.00%	50.00%	50.00%	0.00%	0.00%
31-39	8.33%	50.00%	41.67%	0.00%	0.00%
40-49	29.17%	37.50%	29.17%	4.17%	0.00%
50-59	17.50%	47.50%	25.00%	10.00%	0.00%
60 or over	27.03%	35.14%	29.73%	2.70%	5.41%

40

Table 1.61:   Rate your level of satisfaction concerning the expertise of library subject specialists in your field at your college's medical library. Broken out by gender.

Gender	Highly Satisfied	Satisfied	Somewhat Satisfied	Dissatisfied	Highly Dissatisfied
Male	20.55%	45.21%	26.03%	5.48%	2.74%
Female	23.81%	35.71%	35.71%	4.76%	0.00%

Table 1.62:   Rate your level of satisfaction concerning the expertise of library subject specialists in your field at your college's medical library. Broken out by annual personal income.

Annual Personal Income	Highly Satisfied	Satisfied	Somewhat Satisfied	Dissatisfied	Highly Dissatisfied
Less than $60,000	0.00%	100.00%	0.00%	0.00%	0.00%
$60,000 to $85,000	23.08%	23.08%	53.85%	0.00%	0.00%
$85,000 to $125,000	25.93%	29.63%	40.74%	0.00%	3.70%
$125,000 to 200,000	29.03%	48.39%	12.90%	6.45%	3.23%
More than $200,000	13.16%	52.63%	26.32%	7.89%	0.00%

Table 1.63:   Rate your level of satisfaction concerning the expertise of library subject specialists in your field at your college's medical library. Broken out by tenure status.

Tenure Status	Highly Satisfied	Satisfied	Somewhat Satisfied	Dissatisfied	Highly Dissatisfied
Tenured	16.67%	47.22%	33.33%	2.78%	0.00%
Not tenured but on a tenure track	8.33%	58.33%	33.33%	0.00%	0.00%
Not tenured and not on a tenure track	26.87%	35.82%	26.87%	7.46%	2.99%

Table 1.64: Rate your level of satisfaction concerning the expertise of library subject specialists in your field at your college's medical library. Broken out by main field of medical research.

Main Field of Medical Research	Highly Satisfied	Satisfied	Somewhat Satisfied	Dissatisfied	Highly Dissatisfied
Neuroscience, Psychiatry, and Psychology	21.87%	43.75%	28.12%	6.25%	0.00%
Immunology, Biochemistry, Infectious Diseases, and Microbiology	20.00%	45.00%	25.00%	5.00%	5.00%
Surgery and Anesthesiology	11.11%	44.44%	44.44%	0.00%	0.00%
Imaging, Pathology, Physiology, and Endocrinology	16.67%	41.67%	33.33%	0.00%	8.33%
Public Health, Emergency Medicine, and Family Practice & Pediatrics	38.89%	38.89%	16.67%	5.56%	0.00%
Cancer and Oncology	42.86%	14.29%	42.86%	0.00%	0.00%
Cardiology	12.50%	50.00%	25.00%	12.50%	0.00%
Urology, Nephrology, OBGYN, and Otolaryngology	0.00%	44.44%	44.44%	11.11%	0.00%

Question Nine: Rate your level of satisfaction concerning the quality and depth of the information technology available at your college's medical library.

Table 1.65: Rate your level of satisfaction concerning the quality and depth of the information technology available at your college's medical library.

	Highly Satisfied	Satisfied	Somewhat Satisfied	Dissatisfied	Highly Dissatisfied
Entire Sample	26.72%	50.86%	17.24%	5.17%	0.00%

Table 1.66: Rate your level of satisfaction concerning the quality and depth of the information technology available at your college's medical library. Broken out by country.

Country	Highly Satisfied	Satisfied	Somewhat Satisfied	Dissatisfied	Highly Dissatisfied
USA	26.21%	49.51%	18.45%	5.83%	0.00%
Other	30.77%	61.54%	7.69%	0.00%	0.00%

Table 1.67: Rate your level of satisfaction concerning the quality and depth of the information technology available at your college's medical library. Broken out by public or private college status.

Type of College	Highly Satisfied	Satisfied	Somewhat Satisfied	Dissatisfied	Highly Dissatisfied
Public	26.74%	54.65%	13.95%	4.65%	0.00%
Private	26.67%	40.00%	26.67%	6.67%	0.00%

Table 1.68: Rate your level of satisfaction concerning the quality and depth of the information technology available at your college's medical library. Broken out by age of participant.

Age	Highly Satisfied	Satisfied	Somewhat Satisfied	Dissatisfied	Highly Dissatisfied
30 or under	50.00%	0.00%	50.00%	0.00%	0.00%
31-39	7.69%	84.62%	7.69%	0.00%	0.00%
40-49	33.33%	45.83%	20.83%	0.00%	0.00%
50-59	24.39%	48.78%	14.63%	12.20%	0.00%
60 or over	30.56%	47.22%	19.44%	2.78%	0.00%

Table 1.69: Rate your level of satisfaction concerning the quality and depth of the information technology available at your college's medical library. Broken out by gender.

Gender	Highly Satisfied	Satisfied	Somewhat Satisfied	Dissatisfied	Highly Dissatisfied
Male	27.40%	50.68%	16.44%	5.48%	0.00%
Female	25.58%	51.16%	18.60%	4.65%	0.00%

Table 1.70: Rate your level of satisfaction concerning the quality and depth of the information technology available at your college's medical library. Broken out by annual personal income.

Annual Personal Income	Highly Satisfied	Satisfied	Somewhat Satisfied	Dissatisfied	Highly Dissatisfied
Less than $60,000	0.00%	0.00%	100.00%	0.00%	0.00%
$60,000 to $85,000	14.29%	64.29%	14.29%	7.14%	0.00%
$85,000 to $125,000	40.74%	29.63%	29.63%	0.00%	0.00%
$125,000 to 200,000	35.48%	45.16%	12.90%	6.45%	0.00%
More than $200,000	15.38%	69.23%	10.26%	5.13%	0.00%

Table 1.71: Rate your level of satisfaction concerning the quality and depth of the information technology available at your college's medical library. Broken out by tenure status.

Tenure Status	Highly Satisfied	Satisfied	Somewhat Satisfied	Dissatisfied	Highly Dissatisfied
Tenured	17.14%	62.86%	17.14%	2.86%	0.00%
Not tenured but on a tenure track	23.08%	69.23%	7.69%	0.00%	0.00%
Not tenured and not on a tenure track	32.35%	41.18%	19.12%	7.35%	0.00%

Table 1.72:   Rate your level of satisfaction concerning the quality and depth of the information technology available at your college's medical library. Broken out by main field of medical research.

Main Field of Medical Research	Highly Satisfied	Satisfied	Somewhat Satisfied	Dissatisfied	Highly Dissatisfied
Neuroscience, Psychiatry, and Psychology	15.15%	60.61%	18.18%	6.06%	0.00%
Immunology, Biochemistry, Infectious Diseases, and Microbiology	25.00%	50.00%	20.00%	5.00%	0.00%
Surgery and Anesthesiology	25.00%	50.00%	25.00%	0.00%	0.00%
Imaging, Pathology, Physiology, and Endocrinology	25.00%	41.67%	25.00%	8.33%	0.00%
Public Health, Emergency Medicine, and Family Practice & Pediatrics	55.56%	33.33%	5.56%	5.56%	0.00%
Cancer and Oncology	28.57%	71.43%	0.00%	0.00$	0.00$
Cardiology	37.50%	25.00%	25.00%	12.50%	0.00%

Chapter Two: Library Spending

Question Ten: Imagine yourself running your college library and subject to its budget constraints. Do you think the library should incease spending on additional computer workstations and other advance hardware technologies?

Table 2.1: Imagine yourself running your college library and subject to its budget constraints. Do you think the library should increase spending on additional computer workstations and other advanced hardware technologies?

	Yes	No
Entire Sample	25.53%	74.47%

Table 2.2: Imagine yourself running your college library and subject to its budget constraints. Do you think the library should increase spending on additional computer workstations and other advanced hardware technologies? Broken out by country.

Country	Yes	No
USA	25.78%	74.22%
Other	23.08%	76.92%

Table 2.3: Imagine yourself running your college library and subject to its budget constraints. Do you think the library should increase spending on additional computer workstations and other advanced hardware technologies? Broken out by public or private college status.

Type of College	Yes	No
Public	24.76%	75.24%
Private	27.78%	72.22%

Table 2.4: Imagine yourself running your college library and subject to its budget constraints. Do you think the library should increase spending on additional computer workstations and other advanced hardware technologies? Broken out by age of participant.

Age	Yes	No
30 or under	0.00%	100.00%
31-39	5.88%	94.12%
40-49	17.24%	82.76%
50-59	28.00%	72.00%
60 or over	37.21%	62.79%

Table 2.5: Imagine yourself running your college library and subject to its budget constraints. Do you think the library should increase spending on additional computer workstations and other advanced hardware technologies? Broken out by gender.

Gender	Yes	No
Male	26.44%	73.56%
Female	24.07%	75.93%

Table 2.6: Imagine yourself running your college library and subject to its budget constraints. Do you think the library should increase spending on additional computer workstations and other advanced hardware technologies? Broken out by annual personal income.

Annual Personal Income	Yes	No
Less than $60,000	0.00%	100.00%
$60,000 to $85,000	17.65%	82.35%
$85,000 to $125,000	21.21%	78.79%
$125,000 to 200,000	12.82%	87.18%
More than $200,000	41.30%	58.70%

Table 2.7: Imagine yourself running your college library and subject to its budget constraints. Do you think the library should increase spending on additional computer workstations and other advanced hardware technologies? Broken out by tenure status.

Tenure Status	Yes	No
Tenured	34.04%	65.96%
Not tenured but on a tenure track	11.76%	88.24%
Not tenured and not on a tenure track	23.38%	76.62%

Table 2.8: Imagine yourself running your college library and subject to its budget constraints. Do you think the library should increase spending on additional computer workstations and other advanced hardware technologies? Broken out by main field of medical research.

Main Field of Medical Research	Yes	No
Neuroscience, Psychiatry, and Psychology	37.84%	62.16%
Immunology, Biochemistry, Infectious Diseases, and Microbiology	17.39%	82.61%
Surgery and Anesthesiology	36.36%	63.64%
Imaging, Pathology, Physiology, and Endocrinology	14.29%	85.71%
Public Health, Emergency Medicine, and Family Practice & Pediatrics	21.74%	78.26%
Cancer and Oncology	36.36%	63.64%
Cardiology	10.00%	90.00%
Urology, Nephrology, OBGYN, and Otolaryngology	18.18%	81.82%

Question Eleven: Imagine yourself running your college library and subject to its budget constraints. Do you think the library should increase spending on journal subscriptions?

Table 2.9: Imagine yourself running your college library and subject to its budget constraints. Do you think the library should increase spending on journal subscriptions?

	Yes	No
Entire Sample	58.87%	41.13%

Table 2.10: Imagine yourself running your college library and subject to its budget constraints. Do you think the library should increase spending on journal subscriptions? Broken out by country.

Country	Yes	No
USA	56.25%	43.75%
Other	84.62%	15.38%

Table 2.11: Imagine yourself running your college library and subject to its budget constraints. Do you think the library should increase spending on journal subscriptions? Broken out by public or private college status.

Type of College	Yes	No
Public	58.10%	41.90%
Private	61.11%	38.89%

Table 2.12: Imagine yourself running your college library and subject to its budget constraints. Do you think the library should increase spending on journal subscriptions? Broken out by age of participant.

Age	Yes	No
30 or under	50.00%	50.00%
31-39	76.47%	23.53%
40-49	58.62%	41.38%
50-59	60.00%	40.00%
60 or over	51.16%	48.84%

Table 2.13: Imagine yourself running your college library and subject to its budget constraints. Do you think the library should increase spending on journal subscriptions? Broken out by gender.

Gender	Yes	No
Male	56.32%	43.68%
Female	62.96%	37.04%

Table 2.14: Imagine yourself running your college library and subject to its budget constraints. Do you think the library should increase spending on journal subscriptions? Broken out by annual personal income.

Annual Personal Income	Yes	No
Less than $60,000	100.00%	0.00%
$60,000 to $85,000	76.47%	23.53%
$85,000 to $125,000	63.64%	36.36%
$125,000 to $200,000	58.97%	41.03%
More than $200,000	47.83%	52.17%

Table 2.15: Imagine yourself running your college library and subject to its budget constraints. Do you think the library should increase spending on journal subscriptions? Broken out by tenure status.

Tenure Status	Yes	No
Tenured	61.70%	38.30%
Not tenured but on a tenure track	70.59%	29.41%
Not tenured and not on a tenure track	54.55%	45.45%

Table 2.16: Imagine yourself running your college library and subject to its budget constraints. Do you think the library should increase spending on journal subscriptions? Broken out by main field of medical research.

Main Field of Medical Research	Yes	No
Neuroscience, Psychiatry, and Psychology	56.76%	43.24%
Immunology, Biochemistry, Infectious Diseases, and Microbiology	60.87%	39.13%
Surgery and Anesthesiology	81.82%	18.18%
Imaging, Pathology, Physiology, and Endocrinology	57.14%	42.86%
Public Health, Emergency Medicine, and Family Practice & Pediatrics	52.17%	47.83%
Cancer and Oncology	45.45%	54.55%
Cardiology	50.00%	50.00%
Urology, Nephrology, OBGYN, and Otolaryngology	81.82%	18.18%

Question Twelve: Imagine yourself running your college library and subject to its budget constraints. Do you think the library should increase spending on traditional print books?

Table 2.17: Imagine yourself running your college library and subject to its budget constraints. Do you think the library should increase spending on traditional print books?

	Yes	No
Entire Sample	7.80%	92.20%

Table 2.18: Imagine yourself running your college library and subject to its budget constraints. Do you think the library should increase spending on traditional print books? Broken out by country.

Country	Yes	No
USA	7.81%	92.19%
Other	7.69%	92.31%

Table 2.19: Imagine yourself running your college library and subject to its budget constraints. Do you think the library should increase spending on traditional print books? Broken out by public or private college status.

Type of College	Yes	No
Public	5.71%	94.29%
Private	13.89%	86.11%

Table 2.20: Imagine yourself running your college library and subject to its budget constraints. Do you think the library should increase spending on traditional print books? Broken out by age of participant.

Age	Yes	No
30 or under	0.00%	100.00%
31-39	0.00%	100.00%
40-49	3.45%	96.55%
50-59	8.00%	92.00%
60 or over	13.95%	86.05%

Table 2.21: Imagine yourself running your college library and subject to its budget constraints. Do you think the library should increase spending on traditional print books? Broken out by gender.

Gender	Yes	No
Male	9.20%	90.80%
Female	5.56%	94.44%

Table 2.22: Imagine yourself running your college library and subject to its budget constraints. Do you think the library should increase spending on traditional print books? Broken out by annual personal income.

Annual Personal Income	Yes	No
Less than $60,000	0.00%	100.00%
$60,000 to $85,000	11.76%	88.24%
$85,000 to $125,000	12.12%	87.88%
$125,000 to 200,000	5.13%	94.87%
More than $200,000	6.52%	93.48%

Table 2.23: Imagine yourself running your college library and subject to its budget constraints. Do you think the library should increase spending on traditional print books? Broken out by tenure status.

Tenure Status	Yes	No
Tenured	10.64%	89.36%
Not tenured but on a tenure track	0.00%	100.00%
Not tenured and not on a tenure track	7.79%	92.21%

Table 2.24: Imagine yourself running your college library and subject to its budget constraints. Do you think the library should increase spending on traditional print books? Broken out by main field of medical research.

Main Field of Medical Research	Yes	No
Neuroscience, Psychiatry, and Psychology	2.70%	97.30%
Immunology, Biochemistry, Infectious Diseases, and Microbiology	21.74%	78.26%
Surgery and Anesthesiology	0.00%	100.00%
Imaging, Pathology, Physiology, and Endocrinology	21.43%	78.57%
Public Health, Emergency Medicine, and Family Practice & Pediatrics	4.35%	95.65%
Cancer and Oncology	9.09%	90.91%
Cardiology	0.00%	100.00%
Urology, Nephrology, OBGYN, and Otolaryngology	0.00%	100.00%

Question Thirteen: Imagine yourself running your college library and subject to its budget constraints. Do you think the library should increase spending on e-books?

Table 2.25: Imagine yourself running your college library and subject to its budget constraints. Do you think the library should increase spending on e-books?

	Yes	No
Entire Sample	35.46%	64.54%

Table 2.26: Imagine yourself running your college library and subject to its budget constraints. Do you think the library should increase spending on e-books? Broken out by country.

Country	Yes	No
USA	34.38%	65.63%
Other	46.15%	53.85%

Table 2.27: Imagine yourself running your college library and subject to its budget constraints. Do you think the library should increase spending on e-books? Broken out by public or private college status.

Type of College	Yes	No
Public	38.10%	61.90%
Private	27.78%	72.22%

Table 2.28: Imagine yourself running your college library and subject to its budget constraints. Do you think the library should increase spending on e-books? Broken out by age of participant.

Age	Yes	No
30 or under	0.00%	100.00%
31-39	29.41%	70.59%
40-49	17.24%	82.76%
50-59	50.00%	50.00%
60 or over	34.88%	65.12%

Table 2.29: Imagine yourself running your college library and subject to its budget constraints. Do you think the library should increase spending on e-books? Broken out by gender.

Gender	Yes	No
Male	33.33%	66.67%
Female	38.89%	61.11%

Table 2.30: Imagine yourself running your college library and subject to its budget constraints. Do you think the library should increase spending on e-books? Broken out by annual personal income.

Annual Personal Income	Yes	No
Less than $60,000	0.00%	100.00%
$60,000 to $85,000	29.41%	70.59%
$85,000 to $125,000	39.39%	60.61%
$125,000 to 200,000	33.33%	66.67%
More than $200,000	34.78%	65.22%

Table 2.31: Imagine yourself running your college library and subject to its budget constraints. Do you think the library should increase spending on e-books? Broken out by tenure status.

Tenure Status	Yes	No
Tenured	46.81%	53.19%
Not tenured but on a tenure track	5.88%	94.12%
Not tenured and not on a tenure track	35.06%	64.94%

Table 2.32: Imagine yourself running your college library and subject to its budget constraints. Do you think the library should increase spending on e-books? Broken out by main field of medical research.

Main Field of Medical Research	Yes	No
Neuroscience, Psychiatry, and Psychology	35.14%	64.86%
Immunology, Biochemistry, Infectious Diseases, and Microbiology	30.43%	69.57%
Surgery and Anesthesiology	36.36%	63.64%
Imaging, Pathology, Physiology, and Endocrinology	42.86%	57.14%
Public Health, Emergency Medicine, and Family Practice & Pediatrics	34.78%	65.22%
Cancer and Oncology	36.36%	63.64%
Cardiology	60.00%	40.00%
Urology, Nephrology, OBGYN, and Otolaryngology	18.18%	81.82%

Question Fourteen: Imagine yourself running your college library and subject to its budget constraints. Do you think the library should increase spending on librarians?

Table 2.33: Imagine yourself running your college library and subject to its budget constraints. Do you think the library should increase spending on librarians?

	Yes	No
Entire Sample	14.18%	85.82%

Table 2.34: Imagine yourself running your college library and subject to its budget constraints. Do you think the library should increase spending on librarians? Broken out by country.

Country	Yes	No
USA	13.28%	86.72%
Other	23.08%	76.92%

Table 2.35: Imagine yourself running your college library and subject to its budget constraints. Do you think the library should increase spending on librarians? Broken out by public or private college status.

Type of College	Yes	No
Public	12.38%	87.62%
Private	19.44%	80.56%

Table 2.36: Imagine yourself running your college library and subject to its budget constraints. Do you think the library should increase spending on librarians? Broken out by age of participant.

Age	Yes	No
30 or under	0.00%	100.00%
31-39	11.76%	88.24%
40-49	10.34%	89.66%
50-59	10.00%	90.00%
60 or over	23.26%	76.74%

Table 2.37:   Imagine yourself running your college library and subject to its budget constraints. Do you think the library should increase spending on librarians? Broken out by gender.

Gender	Yes	No
Male	10.34%	89.66%
Female	20.37%	79.63%

Table 2.38:   Imagine yourself running your college library and subject to its budget constraints. Do you think the library should increase spending on librarians? Broken out by annual personal income.

Annual Personal Income	Yes	No
Less than $60,000	0.00%	100.00%
$60,000 to $85,000	41.18%	58.82%
$85,000 to $125,000	18.18%	81.82%
$125,000 to 200,000	7.69%	92.31%
More than $200,000	8.70%	91.30%

Table 2.39:   Imagine yourself running your college library and subject to its budget constraints. Do you think the library should increase spending on librarians? Broken out by tenure status.

Tenure Status	Yes	No
Tenured	6.38%	93.62%
Not tenured but on a tenure track	11.76%	88.24%
Not tenured and not on a tenure track	19.48%	80.52%

Table 2.40: Imagine yourself running your college library and subject to its budget constraints. Do you think the library should increase spending on librarians? Broken out by main field of medical research.

Main Field of Medical Research	Yes	No
Neuroscience, Psychiatry, and Psychology	13.51%	86.49%
Immunology, Biochemistry, Infectious Diseases, and Microbiology	13.04%	86.96%
Surgery and Anesthesiology	9.09%	90.91%
Imaging, Pathology, Physiology, and Endocrinology	28.57%	71.43%
Public Health, Emergency Medicine, and Family Practice & Pediatrics	13.04%	86.96%
Cancer and Oncology	27.27%	72.73%
Cardiology	10.00%	90.00%
Urology, Nephrology, OBGYN, and Otolaryngology	0.00%	100.00%

Question Fifteen: Imagine yourself running your college library and subject to its budget constraints. Do you think the library should increase spending on better facilities?

Table 2.41: Imagine yourself running your college library and subject to its budget constraints. Do you think the library should incrase spending on better facilities?

	Yes	No
Entire Sample	7.80%	92.20%

Table 2.42: Imagine yourself running your college library and subject to its budget constraints. Do you think the library should incrase spending on better facilities? Broken out by country.

Country	Yes	No
USA	8.59%	91.41%
Other	0.00%	100.00%

Table 2.43: Imagine yourself running your college library and subject to its budget constraints. Do you think the library should incrase spending on better facilities? Broken out by public or private college status.

Type of College	Yes	No
Public	6.67%	93.33%
Private	11.11%	88.89%

Table 2.44: Imagine yourself running your college library and subject to its budget constraints. Do you think the library should incrase spending on better facilities? Broken out by age of participant.

Age	Yes	No
30 or under	50.00%	50.00%
31-39	5.88%	94.12%
40-49	6.90%	93.10%
50-59	8.00%	92.00%
60 or over	6.98%	93.02%

Table 2.45:   Imagine yourself running your college library and subject to its budget constraints. Do you think the library should incrase spending on better facilities? Broken out by gender.

Gender	Yes	No
Male	10.34%	89.66%
Female	3.70%	96.30%

Table 2.46:   Imagine yourself running your college library and subject to its budget constraints. Do you think the library should incrase spending on better facilities? Broken out by annual personal income.

Annual Personal Income	Yes	No
Less than $60,000	0.00%	100.00%
$60,000 to $85,000	5.88%	94.12%
$85,000 to $125,000	12.12%	87.88%
$125,000 to 200,000	2.56%	97.44%
More than $200,000	8.70%	91.30%

Table 2.47:   Imagine yourself running your college library and subject to its budget constraints. Do you think the library should incrase spending on better facilities? Broken out by tenure status.

Tenure Status	Yes	No
Tenured	4.26%	95.74%
Not tenured but on a tenure track	5.88%	94.12%
Not tenured and not on a tenure track	10.39%	89.61%

Table 2.48: Imagine yourself running your college library and subject to its budget constraints. Do you think the library should incrase spending on better facilities? Broken out by main field of medical research.

Main Field of Medical Research	Yes	No
Neuroscience, Psychiatry, and Psychology	5.41%	94.59%
Immunology, Biochemistry, Infectious Diseases, and Microbiology	0.00%	100.00%
Surgery and Anesthesiology	9.09%	90.91%
Imaging, Pathology, Physiology, and Endocrinology	14.29%	85.71%
Public Health, Emergency Medicine, and Family Practice & Pediatrics	17.39%	82.61%
Cancer and Oncology	9.09%	90.91%
Cardiology	10.00%	90.00%
Urology, Nephrology, OBGYN, and Otolaryngology	0.00%	100.00%

Chapter Three: Databases

Question Sixteen: Evaluate the range and quality of databases available at your institution's medical library.

Table 3.1:   Evaluate the range and quality of databases available at your institution's medical library.

	Excellent	Good	Acceptable	Poor
Entire Sample	46.83%	38.10%	14.29%	0.79%

Table 3.2:   Evaluate the range and quality of databases available at your institution's medical library. Broken out by country.

Country	Excellent	Good	Acceptable	Poor
USA	45.61%	38.60%	14.91%	0.88%
Other	58.33%	33.33%	8.33%	0.00%

Table 3.3:   Evaluate the range and quality of databases available at your institution's medical library. Broken out by public or private college status.

Type of College	Excellent	Good	Acceptable	Poor
Public	48.94%	36.17%	14.89%	0.00%
Private	40.63%	43.75%	12.50%	3.13%

Table 3.4:   Evaluate the range and quality of databases available at your institution's medical library. Broken out by age of participant.

Age	Excellent	Good	Acceptable	Poor
30 or under	0.00%	0.00%	100.00%	0.00%
31-39	57.14%	42.86%	0.00%	0.00%
40-49	50.00%	33.33%	16.67%	0.00%
50-59	44.68%	36.17%	17.02%	2.13%
60 or over	45.00%	42.50%	12.50%	0.00%

Table 3.5: Evaluate the range and quality of databases available at your institution's medical library. Broken out by gender.

Gender	Excellent	Good	Acceptable	Poor
Male	48.68%	34.21%	15.79%	1.32%
Female	44.00%	44.00%	12.00%	0.00%

Table 3.6: Evaluate the range and quality of databases available at your institution's medical library. Broken out by annual personal income.

Annual Personal Income	Excellent	Good	Acceptable	Poor
Less than $60,000	0.00%	100.00%	0.00%	0.00%
$60,000 to $85,000	25.00%	56.25%	18.75%	0.00%
$85,000 to $125,000	50.00%	40.00%	10.00%	0.00%
$125,000 to 200,000	55.88%	26.47%	17.65%	0.00%
More than $200,000	45.00%	37.50%	15.00%	2.50%

Table 3.7: Evaluate the range and quality of databases available at your institution's medical library. Broken out by tenure status.

Tenure Status	Excellent	Good	Acceptable	Poor
Tenured	42.86%	42.86%	11.90%	2.38%
Not tenured but on a tenure track	58.33%	16.67%	25.00%	0.00%
Not tenured and not on a tenure track	47.22%	38.89%	13.89%	0.00%

Table 3.8: Evaluate the range and quality of databases available at your institution's medical library. Broken out by main field of medical research.

Main Field of Medical Research	Excellent	Good	Acceptable	Poor
Neuroscience, Psychiatry, and Psychology	48.48%	36.36%	15.15%	0.00%
Immunology, Biochemistry, Infectious Diseases, and Microbiology	34.78%	43.48%	21.74%	0.00%
Surgery and Anesthesiology	44.44%	33.33%	22.22%	0.00%
Imaging, Pathology, Physiology, and Endocrinology	45.45%	54.55%	0.00%	0.00%
Public Health, Emergency Medicine, and Family Practice & Pediatrics	57.14%	33.33%	9.52%	0.00%
Cancer and Oncology	36.36%	45.45%	18.18%	0.00%
Cardiology	66.67%	33.33%	0.00%	0.00%
Urology, Nephrology, OBGYN, and Otolaryngology	44.44%	22.22%	22.22%	11.11%

Question Seventeen: Evaluate the range and quality of academic journals available at your institution's medical library.

Table 3.9:   Evaluate the range and quality of academic journals available at your institution's medical library.

	Excellent	Good	Acceptable	Poor
Entire Sample	50.00%	30.95%	16.67%	2.38%

Table 3.10:   Evaluate the range and quality of academic journals available at your institution's medical library. Broken out by country.

Country	Excellent	Good	Acceptable	Poor
USA	50.00%	29.82%	17.54%	2.63%
Other	50.00%	41.67%	8.33%	0.00%

Table 3.11:   Evaluate the range and quality of academic journals available at your institution's medical library. Broken out by public or private college status.

Type of College	Excellent	Good	Acceptable	Poor
Public	52.63%	30.53%	16.84%	0.00%
Private	41.94%	32.26%	16.13%	9.68%

Table 3.12:   Evaluate the range and quality of academic journals available at your institution's medical library. Broken out by age of participant.

Age	Excellent	Good	Acceptable	Poor
30 or under	50.00%	0.00%	50.00%	0.00%
31-39	50.00%	50.00%	0.00%	0.00%
40-49	54.17%	33.33%	12.50%	0.00%
50-59	50.00%	23.91%	21.74%	4.35%
60 or over	47.50%	32.50%	17.50%	2.50%

Table 3.13:   Evaluate the range and quality of academic journals available at your institution's medical library. Broken out by gender.

Gender	Excellent	Good	Acceptable	Poor
Male	46.75%	32.47%	18.18%	2.60%
Female	55.10%	28.57%	14.29%	2.04%

Table 3.14: Evaluate the range and quality of academic journals available at your institution's medical library. Broken out by annual personal income.

Annual Personal Income	Excellent	Good	Acceptable	Poor
Less than $60,000	0.00%	100.00%	0.00%	0.00%
$60,000 to $85,000	31.25%	56.25%	12.50%	0.00%
$85,000 to $125,000	53.33%	23.33%	23.33%	0.00%
$125,000 to 200,000	55.88%	23.53%	11.76%	8.82%
More than $200,000	52.50%	30.00%	17.50%	0.00%

Table 3.15: Evaluate the range and quality of academic journals available at your institution's medical library. Broken out by tenure status.

Tenure Status	Excellent	Good	Acceptable	Poor
Tenured	45.24%	35.71%	16.67%	2.38%
Not tenured but on a tenure track	66.67%	8.33%	25.00%	0.00%
Not tenured and not on a tenure track	50.00%	31.94%	15.28%	2.78%

Table 3.16: Evaluate the range and quality of academic journals available at your institution's medical library. Broken out by main field of medical research.

Main Field of Medical Research	Excellent	Good	Acceptable	Poor
Neuroscience, Psychiatry, and Psychology	46.88%	34.37%	15.63%	3.12%
Immunology, Biochemistry, Infectious Diseases, and Microbiology	34.78%	39.13%	21.74%	4.35%
Surgery and Anesthesiology	55.56%	22.22%	22.22%	0.00%
Imaging, Pathology, Physiology, and Endocrinology	50.00%	41.67%	8.33%	0.00%
Public Health, Emergency Medicine, and Family Practice & Pediatrics	52.38%	38.10%	4.76%	4.76%
Cancer and Oncology	45.45%	27.27%	27.27%	0.00%
Cardiology	100.00%	0.00%	0.00%	0.00%
Urology, Nephrology, OBGYN, and Otolaryngology	44.44%	11.11%	44.44%	0.00%

Question Eighteen: Evaluate the availability and quality of instruction in library resources at your institution's medical library.

Table 3.17: Evaluate the availability and quality of instruction in library resources at your institution's medical library.

	Excellent	Good	Acceptable	Poor
Entire Sample	31.93%	42.02%	21.85%	4.20%

Table 3.18: Evaluate the availability and quality of instruction in library resources at your institution's medical library. Broken out by country.

Country	Excellent	Good	Acceptable	Poor
USA	32.41%	39.81%	23.15%	4.63%
Other	27.27%	63.64%	9.09%	0.00%

Table 3.19: Evaluate the availability and quality of instruction in library resources at your institution's medical library. Broken out by public or private college status.

Type of College	Excellent	Good	Acceptable	Poor
Public	26.97%	48.31%	22.47%	2.25%
Private	46.67%	23.33%	20.00%	10.00%

Table 3.20: Evaluate the availability and quality of instruction in library resources at your institution's medical library. Broken out by age of participant.

Age	Excellent	Good	Acceptable	Poor
30 or under	50.00%	0.00%	50.00%	0.00%
31-39	33.33%	58.33%	8.33%	0.00%
40-49	41.67%	20.83%	29.17%	8.33%
50-59	32.56%	39.53%	27.91%	0.00%
60 or over	23.68%	55.26%	13.16%	7.89%

Table 3.21: Evaluate the availability and quality of instruction in library resources at your institution's medical library. Broken out by gender.

Gender	Excellent	Good	Acceptable	Poor
Male	32.43%	41.89%	20.27%	5.41%
Female	31.11%	42.22%	24.44%	2.22%

Table 3.22: Evaluate the availability and quality of instruction in library resources at your institution's medical library. Broken out by annual personal income.

Annual Personal Income	Excellent	Good	Acceptable	Poor
Less than $60,000	0.00%	0.00%	100.00%	0.00%
$60,000 to $85,000	20.00%	53.33%	26.67%	0.00%
$85,000 to $125,000	42.86%	32.14%	21.43%	3.57%
$125,000 to 200,000	41.18%	32.35%	26.47%	0.00%
More than $200,000	21.62%	51.35%	16.22%	10.81%

Table 3.23: Evaluate the availability and quality of instruction in library resources at your institution's medical library. Broken out by tenure status.

Tenure Status	Excellent	Good	Acceptable	Poor
Tenured	17.95%	58.97%	23.08%	0.00%
Not tenured but on a tenure track	40.00%	20.00%	40.00%	0.00%
Not tenured and not on a tenure track	38.57%	35.71%	18.57%	7.14%

Table 3.24: Evaluate the availability and quality of instruction in library resources at your institution's medical library. Broken out by main field of medical research.

Main Field of Medical Research	Excellent	Good	Acceptable	Poor
Neuroscience, Psychiatry, and Psychology	31.25%	37.50%	25.00%	6.25%
Immunology, Biochemistry, Infectious Diseases, and Microbiology	33.33%	33.33%	33.33%	0.00%
Surgery and Anesthesiology	25.00%	50.00%	25.00%	0.00%
Imaging, Pathology, Physiology, and Endocrinology	36.36%	36.36%	9.09%	18.18%
Public Health, Emergency Medicine, and Family Practice & Pediatrics	38.10%	47.62%	14.29%	0.00%
Cancer and Oncology	27.27%	54.55%	18.18%	0.00%
Cardiology	22.22%	66.67%	11.11%	0.00%
Urology, Nephrology, OBGYN, and Otolaryngology	33.33%	22.22%	33.33%	11.11%

Question Nineteen: Evaluate the speed and quality of interlibrary loan resources at your institution's medical library.

Table 3.25: Evaluate the speed and quality of interlibrary loan resources at your institution's medical library.

	Excellent	Good	Acceptable	Poor
Entire Sample	31.97%	38.52%	22.95%	6.56%

Table 3.26: Evaluate the speed and quality of interlibrary loan resources at your institution's medical library. Broken out by country.

Country	Excellent	Good	Acceptable	Poor
USA	32.73%	35.45%	24.55%	7.27%
Other	25.00%	66.67%	8.33%	0.00%

Table 3.27: Evaluate the speed and quality of interlibrary loan resources at your institution's medical library. Broken out by public or private college status.

Type of College	Excellent	Good	Acceptable	Poor
Public	29.35%	42.39%	23.91%	4.35%
Private	40.00%	26.67%	20.00%	13.33%

Table 3.28: Evaluate the speed and quality of interlibrary loan resources at your institution's medical library. Broken out by age of participant.

Age	Excellent	Good	Acceptable	Poor
30 or under	50.00%	50.00%	0.00%	0.00%
31-39	16.67%	75.00%	8.33%	0.00%
40-49	33.33%	33.33%	29.17%	4.17%
50-59	36.96%	30.43%	21.74%	10.87%
60 or over	28.95%	39.47%	26.32%	5.26%

Table 3.29: Evaluate the speed and quality of interlibrary loan resources at your institution's medical library. Broken out by gender.

Gender	Excellent	Good	Acceptable	Poor
Male	32.00%	41.33%	22.67%	4.00%
Female	31.91%	34.04%	23.40%	10.64%

Table 3.30: Evaluate the speed and quality of interlibrary loan resources at your institution's medical library. Broken out by annual personal income.

Annual Personal Income	Excellent	Good	Acceptable	Poor
Less than $60,000	0.00%	0.00%	100.00%	0.00%
$60,000 to $85,000	26.67%	40.00%	26.67%	6.67%
$85,000 to $125,000	33.33%	40.00%	23.33%	3.33%
$125,000 to 200,000	40.00%	34.29%	17.14%	8.57%
More than $200,000	27.03%	43.24%	21.62%	8.11%

Table 3.31: Evaluate the speed and quality of interlibrary loan resources at your institution's medical library. Broken out by tenure status.

Tenure Status	Excellent	Good	Acceptable	Poor
Tenured	25.64%	41.03%	25.64%	7.69%
Not tenured but on a tenure track	27.27%	54.55%	18.18%	0.00%
Not tenured and not on a tenure track	36.11%	34.72%	22.22%	6.94%

Table 3.32: Evaluate the speed and quality of interlibrary loan resources at your institution's medical library. Broken out by main field of medical research.

Main Field of Medical Research	Excellent	Good	Acceptable	Poor
Neuroscience, Psychiatry, and Psychology	28.12%	34.37%	34.37%	3.12%
Immunology, Biochemistry, Infectious Diseases, and Microbiology	28.57%	28.57%	33.33%	9.52%
Surgery and Anesthesiology	37.50%	37.50%	25.00%	0.00%
Imaging, Pathology, Physiology, and Endocrinology	36.36%	45.45%	0.00%	18.18%
Public Health, Emergency Medicine, and Family Practice & Pediatrics	33.33%	47.62%	9.52%	9.52%
Cancer and Oncology	30.00%	40.00%	30.00%	0.00%
Cardiology	33.33%	55.56%	11.11%	0.00%
Urology, Nephrology, OBGYN, and Otolaryngology	40.00%	30.00%	20.00%	10.00%

Question Twenty: Evaluate the quality of technology instruction available at your institution's medical library.

Table 3.33: Evaluate the quality of technology instruction available at your institution's medical library.

	Excellent	Good	Acceptable	Poor
Entire Sample	30.09%	38.05%	26.55%	5.31%

Table 3.34: Evaluate the quality of technology instruction available at your institution's medical library. Broken out by country.

Country	Excellent	Good	Acceptable	Poor
USA	30.39%	37.25%	26.47%	5.88%
Other	27.27%	45.45%	27.27%	0.00%

Table 3.35: Evaluate the quality of technology instruction available at your institution's medical library. Broken out by public or private college status.

Type of College	Excellent	Good	Acceptable	Poor
Public	24.10%	44.58%	27.71%	3.61%
Private	46.67%	20.00%	23.33%	10.00%

Table 3.36: Evaluate the quality of technology instruction available at your institution's medical library. Broken out by age of participant.

Age	Excellent	Good	Acceptable	Poor
30 or under	0.00%	50.00%	50.00%	0.00%
31-39	18.18%	45.45%	36.36%	0.00%
40-49	43.48%	13.04%	34.78%	8.70%
50-59	35.71%	35.71%	26.19%	2.38%
60 or over	20.00%	54.29%	17.14%	8.57%

Table 3.37: Evaluate the quality of technology instruction available at your institution's medical library. Broken out by gender.

Gender	Excellent	Good	Acceptable	Poor
Male	32.39%	38.03%	25.35%	4.23%
Female	26.19%	38.10%	28.57%	7.14%

Table 3.38: Evaluate the quality of technology instruction available at your institution's medical library. Broken out by annual personal income.

Annual Personal Income	Excellent	Good	Acceptable	Poor
Less than $60,000	0.00%	100.00%	0.00%	0.00%
$60,000 to $85,000	15.38%	38.46%	38.46%	7.69%
$85,000 to $125,000	44.44%	25.93%	22.22%	7.41%
$125,000 to 200,000	38.71%	35.48%	22.58%	3.23%
More than $200,000	21.62%	43.24%	29.73%	5.41%

Table 3.39: Evaluate the quality of technology instruction available at your institution's medical library. Broken out by tenure status.

Tenure Status	Excellent	Good	Acceptable	Poor
Tenured	16.67%	47.22%	33.33%	2.78%
Not tenured but on a tenure track	44.44%	11.11%	44.44%	0.00%
Not tenured and not on a tenure track	35.29%	36.76%	20.59%	7.35%

Table 3.40: Evaluate the quality of technology instruction available at your institution's medical library. Broken out by main field of medical research.

Main Field of Medical Research	Excellent	Good	Acceptable	Poor
Neuroscience, Psychiatry, and Psychology	34.37%	31.25%	28.12%	6.25%
Immunology, Biochemistry, Infectious Diseases, and Microbiology	43.75%	31.25%	18.75%	6.25%
Surgery and Anesthesiology	25.00%	37.50%	37.50%	0.00%
Imaging, Pathology, Physiology, and Endocrinology	27.27%	45.45%	9.09%	18.18%
Public Health, Emergency Medicine, and Family Practice & Pediatrics	35.00%	40.00%	20.00%	5.00%
Cancer and Oncology	11.11%	33.33%	55.56%	0.00%
Cardiology	12.50%	75.00%	12.50%	0.00%
Urology, Nephrology, OBGYN, and Otolaryngology	22.22%	33.33%	44.44%	0.00%

Question Twenty-one: Evaluate the availability and knowledge of library subject specialists in your area at your institution's medical library.

Table 3.41:   Evaluate the availability and knowledge of library subject specialists in your area at your institution's medical library.

	Excellent	Good	Acceptable	Poor
Entire Sample	31.58%	37.72%	24.56%	6.14%

Table 3.42:   Evaluate the availability and knowledge of library subject specialists in your area at your institution's medical library. Broken out by country.

Country	Excellent	Good	Acceptable	Poor
USA	32.04%	38.83%	24.27%	4.85%
Other	27.27%	27.27%	27.27%	18.18%

Table 3.43:   Evaluate the availability and knowledge of library subject specialists in your area at your institution's medical library. Broken out by public or private college status.

Type of College	Excellent	Good	Acceptable	Poor
Public	29.76%	41.67%	23.81%	4.76%
Private	36.67%	26.67%	26.67%	10.00%

Table 3.44:   Evaluate the availability and knowledge of library subject specialists in your area at your institution's medical library. Broken out by age of participant.

Age	Excellent	Good	Acceptable	Poor
30 or under	0.00%	50.00%	50.00%	0.00%
31-39	15.38%	53.85%	30.77%	0.00%
40-49	37.50%	33.33%	20.83%	8.33%
50-59	33.33%	33.33%	25.64%	7.69%
60 or over	33.33%	38.89%	22.22%	5.56%

Table 3.45: Evaluate the availability and knowledge of library subject specialists in your area at your institution's medical library. Broken out by gender.

Gender	Excellent	Good	Acceptable	Poor
Male	32.86%	37.14%	27.14%	2.86%
Female	29.55%	38.64%	20.45%	11.36%

Table 3.46: Evaluate the availability and knowledge of library subject specialists in your area at your institution's medical library. Broken out by annual personal income.

Annual Personal Income	Excellent	Good	Acceptable	Poor
Less than $60,000	0.00%	0.00%	100.00%	0.00%
$60,000 to $85,000	28.57%	50.00%	14.29%	7.14%
$85,000 to $125,000	37.04%	18.52%	29.63%	14.81%
$125,000 to 200,000	33.33%	42.42%	24.24%	0.00%
More than $200,000	25.71%	45.71%	22.86%	5.71%

Table 3.47: Evaluate the availability and knowledge of library subject specialists in your area at your institution's medical library. Broken out by tenure status.

Tenure Status	Excellent	Good	Acceptable	Poor
Tenured	20.00%	40.00%	34.29%	5.71%
Not tenured but on a tenure track	18.18%	45.45%	36.36%	0.00%
Not tenured and not on a tenure track	39.71%	35.29%	17.65%	7.35%

Table 3.48: Evaluate the availability and knowledge of library subject specialists in your area at your institution's medical library. Broken out by main field of medical research.

Main Field of Medical Research	Excellent	Good	Acceptable	Poor
Neuroscience, Psychiatry, and Psychology	31.25%	43.75%	18.75%	6.25%
Immunology, Biochemistry, Infectious Diseases, and Microbiology	23.53%	35.29%	29.41%	11.76%
Surgery and Anesthesiology	33.33%	33.33%	33.33%	0.00%
Imaging, Pathology, Physiology, and Endocrinology	16.67%	41.67%	25.00%	16.67%
Public Health, Emergency Medicine, and Family Practice & Pediatrics	36.84%	42.11%	21.05%	0.00%
Cancer and Oncology	10.00%	40.00%	50.00%	0.00%
Cardiology	62.50%	25.00%	12.50%	0.00%
Urology, Nephrology, OBGYN, and Otolaryngology	50.00%	20.00%	20.00%	10.00%

www.ingramcontent.com/pod-product-compliance
Lightning Source LLC
Chambersburg PA
CBHW081553220326
41598CB00036B/6665